THE ESS

Natural Pet Care

ARTHRITIS

THE ESSENTIAL GUIDE TO

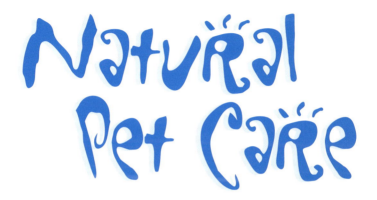

Natural Pet Care

ARTHRITIS

JOAN HUSTACE WALKER

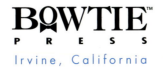

BOWTIE™
PRESS
Irvine, California

Special thanks go to Dr. Nancy Scanlan for freely sharing her expertise in the area of arthritis and for making my job as a writer so easy.   —J. H. W.

Ruth Berman, editor-in-chief
Nick Clemente, special consultant
Book design and layout by Michele Lanci-Altomare
Mike Uyesugi, cover design

Library of Congress Cataloging-in-Publication Data

Walker, Joan Hustace, 1962-
    Arthritis / Joan Hustace Walker.
        p.   cm. -- (Essential guide to natural pet care)
    Includes bibliographical references (p.).
    ISBN 1-889540-33-1 (softcover : alk. paper)
    1. Dogs--Diseases--Alternative treatment. 2. Pets--Diseases-
  -Alternative treatment. 3. Arthritis in animals--Alternative
  treatment. 4. Holistic veterinary medicine. I. Title
    II. Series.
    SF992.A77W25 1999
    636.089'6722--dc21   99-22313
                                                               CIP

BowTie™ Press
3 Burroughs
Irvine, California 92618

Manufactured in the United States of America
10 9 8 7 6 5 4 3 2 1

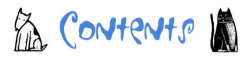

Contents

Arthritis is one of the most common problems seen in older animals. Unfortunately, the two standard conventional veterinary treatments for arthritis, corticosteroids and nonsteroidal anti-inflammatory drugs, have many problems associated with them. These problems are readily acknowledged by the conventional medical community, but many conventional veterinarians don't have any better treatments to offer patients.

Fortunately, arthritis responds extremely well to holistic medicine. Even the conventional veterinary medical

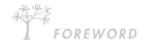
community has begun to recognize the advantages of using more natural treatments, and mainstream pharmaceutical companies are now manufacturing a few natural products for veterinary use. Holistic veterinarians use many methods to treat arthritis, such as acupuncture, chiropractic, homeopathy, herbal medicine, nutritional supplements, massage therapy, and many others, but it is difficult to find one source that discusses all these holistic treatment options. *Arthritis* fills this gap and offers an in-depth discussion of the holistic methods that are effective in treating this disease.

—*Nancy Scanlan, D.V.M.*

What Is Holistic Care?

Holistic care goes by many names: alternative medicine, complementary care, preventive therapy, and environmental medicine, to name a few. Though the exclusive use of holistic veterinary care is uncommon, many holistic therapies are receiving increasing support from the veterinary community. With pet owners and veterinarians seeking less-invasive and gentler means of treating injuries, illnesses, and chronic conditions, holistic care is rapidly gaining popularity across the country and acceptance among an increasing number of health-care professionals.

The term *holistic care* conjures up different images for different people. For some pet owners, it is a viable, working system of veterinary care. For others, it may bring to mind more skeptical images of mystics and healers. In reality, holistic care probably falls somewhere in between these two views. Though many methods are just beginning to undergo clinical trials to prove their efficacy, practitioners have been treating many conditions holistically with recorded success for centuries. Holistic treatments include veterinary chiropractic, acupuncture, supplementation, orthomolecular medicine (curing disease or mental illness by restoring optimum amounts of substances already found in the body), herbs, and homeopathy.

This is not to say that holistic practitioners do not use any conventional methods of treatment. According to the American Holistic Veterinary Medical Association (AHVMA), holistic treatment plans may include conventional Western medical technology (i.e., surgery, drug therapy, and diagnostics such as blood work and X rays). The AHVMA says that in many acute situations such as severe trauma and certain infections, Western medicine often "out performs other methodologies." For this reason, holistic treatments are often referred to as "complementary" medicine, as opposed to "alternative" medicine, in that holistic modalities are used to enhance what conventional medicine has to offer.

THE DIFFERENCES BETWEEN HOLISTIC CARE AND WESTERN MEDICINE

As holistic modalities become more accepted by mainstream medical practitioners, the differences between holistic and conventional medicine will become more difficult to pinpoint. At the current time, however, there are a few basic aspects of holistic care that make it unique from its Western cousin.

Whole Patient vs. Symptoms

One of the key differences between conventional medicine and holistic care is how the practitioner approaches a problem or illness. In conventional medicine, the problem is diagnosed and the symptoms are treated. In holistic medicine, the doctor diagnoses the problem but also attempts to treat the whole animal—not just the symptoms. The veterinarian tries to determine why the infection or illness was able to establish itself and what factors caused the problem in the first place. After a thorough physical, mental, and emotional examination of the animal (which includes a lot of questions for the owner about the pet's environment and temperament), the holistic veterinarian may choose to treat the animal's immune system (by prescribing an herbal remedy and/or a change in diet) and improve the pet's emotional state, perhaps by using flower essences.

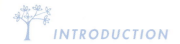

Internal Healing Powers vs. Pharmaceuticals

A large part of holistic care rests in the belief that the body's natural healing powers can be induced, or stimulated, to help the body heal itself. For example, acupuncture has been proven to release endorphins, the body's natural painkillers.

Conventional medicine typically does not call on the body to heal itself but provides medicines that fight the illness for the patient. Some proponents of holistic medicine argue that drugs such as antibiotics do nothing to build up the patient's immunity to subsequent infections and might also have detrimental side effects. (Holistic treatments are generally noted for their gentleness and lack of side effects.) But cases in which a cat or dog needs immediate pain relief or has a horrendous infection, holistic practitioners may use conventional methods or refer the patient to a conventional veterinarian to treat the problem.

Proof

Conventional medicine practices are based on recorded proof that the procedure, therapy, or pharmaceutical works. A treatment can't work just once for one patient. It can't be a theory. The efficacy of the product or treatment must be proven through double-blind studies in which neither the patient, pet owner, or the practitioner knows which patient is receiving the treatment being tested and which patient is receiving the placebo, or sugar pill. There must be clinical trials. There must be oodles of recorded documentation that the treatment actually works every time and all the time.

Holistic medicine is a bit different. Though some therapies such as acupuncture and herbs have been used for thousands of years, there have not been many studies documenting their effectiveness until recently. Research in the areas of acupuncture and chiropractic indicate that these modalities can be used effectively for many conditions. Nutraceuticals (minerals, vitamins, and nutrients) and herbal medicines also are the focus of researchers. Dietary supplements such as glucosamine are being studied for their effects on fortifying cartilage in diseased joints. In the herbal field, some industry members are making an effort to use pharmaceutical-style testing to prove the quality and effectiveness of their products.

As holistic methodologies continue to grow in popularity, it can be assumed that more trials will be performed to explain the *how* and *why* of these successful modalities.

Precision vs. Variation

In conventional medicine, the active ingredients of prescribed medications are administered in precise,

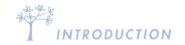

laboratory-controlled dosages. With holistic medicine, practitioners don't have the luxury of knowing the exact potency
of each herb. Just as the melons of one field may be sweet
and those of another have no taste, one crop of herbs may
be potent, while another may be relatively weak. As more
standardization is sought within the industry, the discrepan-
cy in precision between conventional pharmaceuticals and
holistic herbs and supplements will no longer be an issue.

Where Holistic Methods Are Taught

Holistic care is often considered an alternative to conventional medicine because it contains methods of
treatment not frequently taught in medical and veterinary
schools. Basically, as soon as a methodology is taught as
part of the core curriculum for all veterinary teaching hospi-
tals, the methodology is no longer considered alternative
and becomes conventional. Many veterinary colleges are
currently teaching holistic methodologies in addition to conventional medicine. Holistic practitioners expect the number
of schools with alternative medicine courses to grow.

HOW HOLISTIC CARE CAN HELP ARTHRITIC PETS

Instead of being subjected to a regime of anti-inflammatory
medication and eventually cortisone-like drugs and/or

surgery, a severely arthritic pet following a holistic regime receives natural therapeutic treatments that would reduce pain, increase strength and mobility, and slow and stop the progression of the disease—with little or no severe side effects. It is important to understand that at this time no medicine—conventional or holistic—can fully reverse or cure true arthritis once the bony changes have set in. (Diseases that produce symptoms similar to arthritis but are not considered to be true arthritis can be reversed or sometimes cured.) The only treatments available are those that ease pain and slow the progression of the disease.

FINDING A GOOD HOLISTIC VETERINARIAN

As with any medical practice, the outcome of a pre-scribed treatment plan depends on a correct diagnosis, an appropriate plan of care, quality products (i.e., herbs, supplements), and skill. An incorrect diagnosis, the wrong care plan, inferior nutraceuticals, or an inept hand at chiropractic or acupuncture will gain your pet nothing and may even cost your pet her health. As with any profession, there are good practitioners and bad practitioners. Because this field is so new, how can you know if you're taking your pet to a qualified holistic professional?

For starters, check up on the prospective veterinarian's

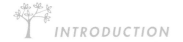

credentials. Is he or she a member of the American Veterinary Medical Association (AVMA), the AHVMA, or the International Veterinary Acupuncture Society (IVAS)? If licensure is required in your state for a veterinarian to practice acupuncture or chiropractic, does this individual have that license?

Also, find out where the veterinarian received his or her holistic training and how many hours were required to train for that particular specialty. For example, 3 hours of chiropractic training does not make a veterinarian an expert in chiropractic technique, but 150 hours of training and five years of practice with yearly postgraduate training probably does.

And, of course, ask people for referrals. Are they happy to extol the virtues of a doctor, or are their answers more guarded? Take note. Then meet with the veterinarian. What is your impression? Does the individual come across as one who goes the extra mile to explain to you what he or she is doing and how a treatment plan will affect your pet, or is it difficult to maintain an open line of communication? Even if the veterinarian is well versed in holistic care, if the two of you can't communicate, you won't be able to tap into his or her expertise.

By taking the time to find a holistic veterinarian who is experienced, skilled, well informed, and communicative, you will be on your way to a solid working relationship that will reward both your pet and you.

What Is Arthritis?

According to one recent study, canine osteoarthritis strikes an estimated one in five adult dogs—or roughly 20 percent of the forty-four million adult dogs in the United States. This same study indicates that dogs most at risk of developing osteoarthritis are large breeds, geriatric dogs, active dogs (e.g., working or sporting dogs), and those with inherited joint abnormalities such as hip or elbow dysplasia.

This study does not represent the whole picture when it comes to pets suffering from arthritis. For one, it doesn't touch on

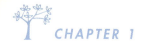

other species, such as cats, who can suffer from chronic arthritic pain, too. Also, the number of pets estimated to have arthritis could be low for the simple reason that pet owners often do not recognize an animal's signs of chronic pain and the pet's arthritis is left untreated (and unreported). The study estimates that more than half of the mild arthritis cases and 44 percent of the moderate cases go untreated. Nearly 20 percent of severe cases receive no veterinary care either.

TYPES OF ARTHRITIS

Though there are more than one hundred diseases that can cause arthritis in pets, true arthritis (as opposed to diseases that cause arthritis-like symptoms) is an inflammation of the joint and can come in many forms, with the two most common being osteoarthritis and rheumatoid arthritis.

Osteoarthritis, the more prevalent of the two, is a degenerative disease that affects joint cartilage, causing it to wear roughly, ulcerate, and in some cases dissolve or disappear, leaving a cushionless bone-on-bone joint. The onset of osteoarthritis can be caused by a developmental or degenerative disease that creates joint instability, which in turn causes the production of painful and destructive bony spurs. Dogs who suffer from hip dysplasia, elbow dysplasia, or other musculoskeletal problems are often at increased risk of developing arthritis as they age. A direct injury that has caused ligament, cartilage, or bone damage to the joint can also increase an animal's risk of developing osteoarthritis. Old age, per se, is not a cause of arthritis, but an older dog who has been very active in life has more opportunities for wear and tear on his joints than his less-active, younger counterparts. Heavy animals put more stress on their joints than do lightweight animals and therefore run a greater risk of developing arthritic joints. Also, chondrodysplastic breeds—those with abnormally short bone growth commonly in the legs, such as dachshunds and basset hounds—often have unstable disks in their backs or necks, which can lead to arthritis.

Rheumatoid arthritis is not a wear-and-tear disease but rather a systemic, autoimmune disease that affects the animal's entire body. Rheumatoid arthritis causes the body's own immune system to attack healthy joint tissue, causing inflammation and joint damage. Fortunately, this type of arthritis is not common in dogs or cats.

There are no cures for either osteoarthritis or rheumatoid arthritis, but there are many holistic treatments that can slow the progression of the disease and provide pain relief to a suffering pet.

THE DEGENERATIVE CYCLE

Part of the vicious cycle of arthritis is that the afflicted animal shows no sign of pain until real joint damage has been achieved. Joints consist of three basic parts: the cartilage that covers the bone, the joint capsule, and the synovial fluid. The start of arthritis generally occurs with an injury to the joint cartilage. Cartilage is living tissue that forms a cushion for the stresses placed on the joint. Cartilage has no nerves, so damage to joint cartilage is not felt by the animal. The joint capsule encloses the joint and contains a thin membrane, called a synovial membrane. The joint capsule produces the third structure of the joint: synovial fluid. This fluid fills the joint cavity, lubricating, nourishing, and cleaning the joint cartilage.

When the joint cartilage is damaged, the tissues release enzymes that erode the cartilage itself and break down the synovial fluid. A small injury to the cartilage can grow into a larger loss of cartilage and synovial fluid as the degenerative cycle continues, but it is not until the injury reaches the joint capsule or the bone itself that the first signs of arthritic pain begin to appear.

DOES YOUR PET HAVE ARTHRITIS?

Though a veterinarian can sometimes diagnose arthritis clinically with a hands-on examination, the only absolute way to diagnose arthritis is with an X ray of the joint.

The signs of arthritic pain can be quite subtle among more stoic pets, so the pet owner plays a critical part in noticing that his or her pet is suffering, enabling the veterinarian to make a diagnosis and begin treatment. Since the disease is degenerative, it is important that an accurate diagnosis is made as early as possible and that immediate treatment is begun.

Mild arthritic pain: Some dogs and cats naturally have a high tolerance for pain and may mask their pain. But most pets with mild cases of arthritis exhibit some stiffness or lameness, particularly when transitioning from a prone position to an upright position, or perhaps when walking after a long period of rest. The animal may also show reluctance walking up or down stairs. The arthritic joints may be somewhat painful to the touch. Though still in the early stages, a mild case of arthritis shows up on an X ray.

Moderate arthritic pain: At the moderate stage a pet may have already lost up to 50 percent of his natural range of motion, resulting in a shortened gait. A dog or cat may yip or otherwise vocalize his pain when rising, jumping into a car, or similarly aggravating the affected joints. A tall dog may choose to lie down while eating out of his food bowl. A cat may uncharacteristically choose to lie on hot pavement on a warm day in an attempt to provide comfort to his aching joints. Some pets may lick the painful joint, and most will let owners know they are in pain when the arthritic joint is palpated. Generally, the degeneration found in the joints is fairly well pronounced in X rays and easily diagnosed.

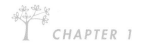 Severe arthritic pain: At the severe stage, most owners can tell that their pet is in intense pain. Walking is extremely difficult for the pet and the preferred position is lying down. Even in this position, the pet may cry out often because the joints hurt with the slightest movement. He may show behavioral changes too; growling, whining, and snapping are not uncommon displays in arthritic dogs. Arthritic cats may show similar short-tempered, *I'm-in-pain* types of responses, too. X rays at this point show severe degeneration of the joints.

Be aware that some dogs and cats can show all the signs of arthritis (even the severe symptoms) and yet suffer from muscular problems that have nothing to do with true arthritis. In these cases, the X rays will not show signs of arthritis, however if your pet suffers these symptoms and does not have arthritis, he can be helped by some of the same holistic treatments that are used to treat arthritis.

LIVING WITH ARTHRITIS

If your pet is diagnosed with arthritis, the first step your holistic veterinarian most likely will take is to perform a complete physical and mental evaluation to determine the cause or source of your pet's discomfort. The reason for this is that with more than one hundred causes of arthritis, some are diseases that can be treated. Additionally, if the cause of your pet's arthritis is a taxing activity such as catching discs in competition, jumping hurdles in obedience, or performing the fast-paced moves of herding sheep all day, you can prevent further destruction of the joint cartilage by halting activities that stress the joint.

A complete evaluation of your pet gives your veterinarian a better understanding of factors, such as genetics, nutrition, stress, exercise, hygiene, habits (both good and bad), and the dog's living environment, that might be influencing the progression of the disease. With this information, the holistic veterinarian will be better equipped to develop a comprehensive, holistic care plan that will treat all aspects of your pet in the most effective, least invasive, and most healthful manner (with the least amount of side effects) possible.

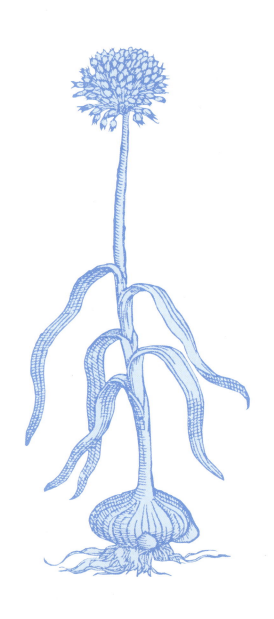

Holistic Therapies

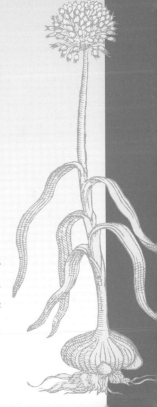

The goal of holistic veterinary care for a patient suffering from arthritis is not only to relieve the animal's pain but also to slow or even stop the progression of the pet's joint degeneration. Though both conventional and holistic medicine practitioners continue to search for a cure or a guarantee of prevention, neither one exists at this time.

Conventional treatment of arthritis involves early intervention and a program of moderate exercise, weight control, cage confinement, and anti-inflammatory drugs.

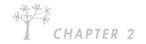

Cortisone-like drugs and surgery may follow. Some complementary methods of treatment, such as polysulfated glycosaminoglycans (PSGAGs), are used by conventional veterinarians. Emerging medical research indicates that PSGAGs thicken joint cartilage and regenerate hyaline cartilage (normal joint cartilage) from abnormal fibrocartilage (a mixture of scar tissue and cartilage that is formed after joint damage).

The problem with some conventional treatment options is that many prescribed drugs have serious side effects. For example, nonsteroidal anti-inflammatory drugs (NSAIDs) can cause stomach ulcers with repeated use and for some patients liver disease, Cushing's syndrome, diabetes, and even a reduced resistance to infections. Those drugs that provide pain relief but do nothing to help correct the joint problem may actually cause more damage as the animal unknowingly stresses the diseased joint while in a pain-free state. Surgery is an invasive procedure and is not without its own inherent risks.

Many pet owners seek holistic veterinary care for its gentle effectiveness. Currently, there are many holistic modalities that can be used to successfully treat arthritis. Because holistic veterinary care is based on the needs of each pet, treatment plans tend to be individualistic. The most commonly used holistic modalities to treat arthritis include acupuncture, chiropractic, herbs, homeo-pathic remedies, and nutritional supplements. A holistic care plan will also include other treatments that owners can supervise at home.

The following is just a small sample of the vast range of holistic treatments available. Depending on your pet's unique situation, your holistic vet may not include a particular modality as part of your pet's treatment plan.

THERAPY # 1
ACUPUNCTURE

Acupuncture has been used for more than three thousand years and remains the primary medical modality for more than 25 percent of the world's human population today, according to the AVMA. It is based on the concept that every animal has energy, *qi* (pronounced "chee"), that flows through the body along channels called meridians. If the flow of energy is not smooth and continuous, diseases can occur. The goal of acupuncture is to unblock the meridians and regain the continuous flow of body energy. This is accomplished by inserting thin needles into meridian points located beneath the skin. With the flow of *qi* regained, the health of the patient is also recovered.

Acupuncture has been credited with increasing an animal's recuperative powers, boosting immunity and

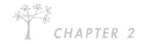

improving mental health. Conventional medicine has determined that when needles are inserted into the acupuncture points, neurotransmitters and neurohormones are stimulated, resulting in the release of the body's natural pain relievers and anti-inflammatory substances. In addition to providing an arthritic pet with instant pain relief, acupuncture can also release muscle spasms around arthritic joints, which increases microcirculation in the joint capsule and joint and slows the degenerative process of cartilage destruction. Boosting the animal's immune system is also important in slowing down the degeneration of joint cartilage—particularly in those pets suffering from rheumatoid arthritis.

Skilled acupuncturists are adept with their needles, and pet owners need not worry about their pets experiencing anything more than mild discomfort during treatment. Unlike an injection, which uses a larger, hollow needle to allow the passage of fluid, an acupuncture needle is very thin and solid. Human patients report very slight sensations as the needle is inserted, with some patients indicating no feeling at all. Amazingly, most pet owners say that their pets are quite calm through the treatments. No anesthesia is necessary for the procedure.

More than thirty states and the District of Columbia license acupuncturists, and eleven more states are drafting or introducing legislation to license acupuncturists as well, reports the National Acupuncture and Oriental Medicine Alliance. Acupuncture is believed to be one of the fastest growing forms of health care in the U.S. It is recognized by the AVMA as "an integral part of veterinary medicine" and is regarded as a "medical procedure under state veterinary practice acts," according to the "Guidelines for Alternative and Complementary Veterinary Medicine," published by the AVMA.

THERAPY #2
CHIROPRACTIC

For dogs and cats with arthritis, range of motion in the afflicted joints is a problem. As the disease progresses, it becomes increasingly difficult for a pet to move with any comfort—and eventually they have difficulty moving at all. Chiropractic treatments can help, say practitioners, by relieving musculoskeletal pain and restoring as much of the pet's range of motion as possible. Restoring movement to a diseased joint also helps retard or halt the progression of the disease. Following the "use it, don't lose it" credo of arthritis sufferers, if an animal is unable to use her joints, the joints generally degrade at a much faster rate than joints that are used and moved moderately.

Chiropractic dates back centuries, but today's form of chiropractic treatment has become accepted only in the

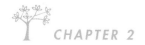

last few decades. Its acceptance among humans is ahead of its use on animals by more than a decade.

Chiropractic is a system of therapy that attempts to restore normal movement and nerve function by releasing abnormal tensions, called chiropractic vertebral subluxations, on the vertebrae. A trauma such as a fall, a chemical imbalance such as an allergic reaction, an emotional response such as sadness, and owner manipulation such as repetitive, sharp obedience corrections are all conditions that can cause an animal to alter her posture and thereby affect her spine. (The pain caused by an arthritic joint can also be a source of a subluxation.) When an animal's spine is affected, the physiological misalignments cause compromised nerve function. This can take the form of additional pain, or it can affect the animal's immune system and organ functions since nerves from the spinal column supply organs and other areas of the body.

The procedure used to correct a subluxation of the spine is called an adjustment. A chiropractic adjustment is a controlled, short-lever, high-velocity, low-amplitude thrust made to the joints (vertebrae) in the spine. The adjustment is performed by hand or with a special instrument. Some veterinarians and chiropractors adjust the entire spine; other practitioners adjust only the area they determine as problematic.

The procedure requires no painkillers nor is it considered to be uncomfortable. It has been reported that an animal may whimper, bark, or bite, when an animal chiropractor adjusts a joint. Often, however, the animal rewards her practitioner with an instant look of gratitude, a yawn, and a stretch.

Pet owners should know that in some states both chiropractors and veterinarians are allowed to adjust animals. In other states, only veterinary chiropractors may work on animals because a dog and cat's physiology is quite different from a human's. If you choose to work with a veterinarian, make sure he or she has received extensive training (one hundred hours or more) and certification from a recognized course such as the one offered by the American Veterinary Chiropractic Association (AVCA). If you're working with a chiropractor who isn't also a vet, it is extremely important that he or she has been trained extensively with animals (preferably certified by the AVCA) and works in concert with your veterinarian.

THERAPY #3
HOMEOPATHY

Homeopathy began in the early 1800s with German physician Samuel Hahnemann, who used the law of similars as

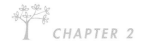

the basis for his development. Hahnemann believed that a disease could be cured by giving a patient a tiny dosage of medicine that produces symptoms similar to the disease in a healthy subject. For example, a dog experiencing nausea might be given a dilute dose (one part to one thousand) of ipecac, which would induce vomiting if given to an animal in full strength.

Homeopathic remedies are usually available in sugar tablets. If your pet won't eat tablets, you can dissolve them in one teaspoon of distilled water. Shake up the solution and use an eyedropper to give the remedy to your pet orally. You can also crush the tablets onto a piece of paper and pour the powder into the animal's cheek.

The most commonly used homeopathic treatment for arthritis is the poison ivy treatment. Poison ivy, or *Rhus toxicodendron,* is often used as a homeopathic remedy for pets suffering from "rusty gate" arthritis, which is pain that is present when an animal first moves but then decreases as the animal gets up and moves about. This homeopathic remedy is also used if a pet tends to have red, inflamed skin.

Another homeopathic remedy called silicea contains extremely diluted silica. Used most frequently for joint and bone diseases that are thought to be inherited, silicea helps pets who do not benefit from increased movement and who suffer even more pain as they move around.

Homeopaths may also recommend remedies to treat the mental aspect of your pet's illness. For example, *Pulsatilla nigricans* may be prescribed for a pet who desires cuddling and attention when ill. *Hekla lava* for pain from bone spurs and *Arnica montana* for muscle soreness are additional remedies sometimes used for arthritic patients.

It is important to note that in homeopathic medicine, doctors rarely prescribe more than one treatment at a time. The reason for this, relates one practitioner, is that a disease may have many layers. As each layer of the disease is treated, a new layer is exposed—often requiring a different treatment. Much of the success of homeopathic medicine lies with the expertise of the practitioner and his or her ability to diagnose the layer of the disease that needs to be treated first.

It is not advisable to give your pet homeopathic remedies without consulting a holistic veterinarian. Cookbook directions for homeopathic dilutions are not as effective as using a treatment that has been specifically prescribed for your pet's unique situation. Homeopathic remedies, though extremely mild, may have implications if used incorrectly. The theory is that any drug with the potential to cure a disease, relieve pain, or otherwise affect the mental or physical health of an animal also has the potential to do damage to an animal if prescribed or used incorrectly.

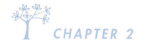

THERAPY #4
HERBAL MEDICINE

Herbs have been used medicinally since at least 5000 B.C. If you take a look at the drugs developed in the last two centuries, many of their origins are from plants, herbs, and flowers. So what separates conventional medicine's use of plants from holistic herbal remedies?

In conventional medicine, the components of a plant are broken down in an attempt to determine what active ingredient creates the desired effect. This chemical is isolated and reproduced in a laboratory. To test the effectiveness of the ingredient, a battery of tests and trials are run before the manufacturers of the drug can apply for Food and Drug Administration (FDA) approval.

Herbal remedies, on the other hand, are not considered to be drugs by the FDA; they are considered to be food products and are not required, at present, to meet the tedious specifications that drugs must pass. Herbal remedies are not broken down into components because many practitioners believe that the whole herb is a more potent remedy than any one particular ingredient contained within the herb.

Herbal remedies do work, but a common complaint among veterinarians is the lack of quality control with some manufacturers. Practitioners warn that not all manufacturers produce consistent, quality products. When quality is lacking, the levels of potency can vary from batch to batch. Therefore, it's important when working with herbs to use only quality products.

In treating arthritis, the benefit of using herbs is that they can be extremely effective (though not as fast acting or as powerful as steroids) and usually have fewer side effects and less dangerous or life-threatening side effects than steroids have.

There are so many herbal remedies that are used successfully to treat arthritic symptoms that to mention them all would be a book in itself. The following are just a few of the herbs that might be prescribed for your pet.

Buckbean *(Menyanthes trifoliata)* and burdock *(Arctium lappa)* can be used to boost the immune system. Lignum vitae *(Guaiacum officinale)* and wild yam *(Dioscorea villosa)* are often successful in reducing painful swelling in and around the arthritic joint. Valerian root *(Valeriana officinalis)*, Jamaican dogwood *(Piscidia erythrina)*, and black cohosh root *(Cimicifuga racemosa)* can act as antispasmodics to reduce muscular tension. White willow bark *(Salix alba)* and yucca *(Yucca schidigera)* are used as analgesics to reduce joint pain, but do not give white willow bark to your cat. Other holistic favorites for treating arthritis include alfalfa *(Medicago sativa)*, cayenne *(Capsicum)*, and meadowsweet *(Filipendula ulmaria)*. Chinese herbal combinations containing multiple herbs commonly

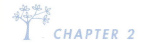

used for arthritis include *Liu Wei Di Huang Wan, Du Huo Jisheng Wan,* and *Chin Koo Tieh Shang Wan.*

Again, as with other gentle holistic treatments, do not give herbal medicines to your pet without the direction and supervision of a holistic veterinarian skilled in herbal medicine. The potency of some herbs can be quite strong and could harm your pet if given inappropriately.

THERAPY #5
NUTRITIONAL SUPPLEMENTS

Good nutrition for an arthritic pet is critical. In addition to prescribing a high-quality diet, many holistic veterinarians often supplement a patient's diet with amino acids, vitamins, minerals, herbs, and other dietary products. As with herbal remedies, some manufacturers produce higher quality supplements than others. Supplements can be harmful if administered inappropriately or at the wrong dosage.

Depending on your pet's diagnosis, your veterinarian may prescribe one or more supplements to be added to your pet's daily diet. The following supplements seem to be most helpful when working with arthritic pets.

Vitamin C: An antioxidant, vitamin C seeks out and destroys free radicals, those annoying molecules that damage proteins, cell membranes, organ cells, and DNA, weakening whatever body part the molecules choose to attack. Vitamin C is water soluble. All water-soluble nutrients are the first to leave the body when it is under stress, so correct levels are difficult to maintain in a pet suffering from stress or severe pain. Holistic practitioners often prescribe large doses of vitamin C to reduce inflammation, improve the immune system, and promote healing.

Vitamin E: Another antioxidant, vitamin E is fat soluble and helps to dilate blood vessels and improve circulation. There has been some serious research on the effects of vitamin E, and studies indicate that it can inhibit inflammation and reduce swelling and pain. Studies also indicate that the natural form of vitamin E is more efficient than the synthetic form. Your veterinarian may prescribe concentrated doses of vitamin E. If so, be aware that it may cause diarrhea in high doses.

Vitamin B complex: Vitamin supplements rich in B complex are often prescribed for animals experiencing psychological problems. Vitamin B complex is believed to help animals cope with stress. The vitamin is water soluble, so it is one of the first, along with vitamin C, to be depleted from a pet suffering pain or stress.

Glucosamine and chondroitin sulfates: Glucosamine, which is made of glucose and an amino acid is a key ingredient in the manufacturing of both cartilage and synovial fluid. It can be derived from mammals (bovine trachea, aorta, and nasal septum), shellfish, sharks, and plants. Glucosamine sulfate is the most active form; recent studies indicate that glucosamine HCl is less effective.

Glucosamine sulfate has shown promise in preventing cartilage degeneration, repairing damaged cartilage, and acting as an anti-inflammatory. Researchers are currently testing the effects of glucosamine on such subjects as dogs, horses, and humans. The substances also have shown promise in causing few if any of the undesirable side effects caused by NSAIDs.

Chondroitin sulfates are long chains of glucosamine units that help prevent enzymes from destroying cartilage. Chondroitin sulfates also help keep water contained within the joint fluid. When glucosamine sulfate is used in concert with chondroitin sulfate, the effect is reported to be synergistic, in that the whole has much greater effect than the sum of either of its parts in stimulating the body to produce cartilage and healthy joint fluid.

Once again, use these supplements only under the direction and supervision of an experienced veterinarian. Though they have shown little if any serious side effects, they should be given in the correct dosage. Also, it is said that the compounds take a while to show effectiveness, so pet owners should be patient.

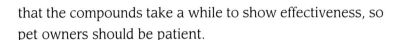 Green-lipped mussels: *Perna canaliculus,* or green-lipped mussels, are a rich source of PSGAGs and work similarly to glucosamine. The use of mussels in holistic treatments is growing and is also attracting the interest of conventional medicine.

Superoxide dismutase (SOD): One of the by-products of inflammation is a group of chemicals known as superoxides. When the superoxides combine with tissues, proteins, and enzymes, they cause more inflammation, which in turn causes the production of more superoxides. Superoxide dismutase is an enzyme that breaks down superoxides into harmless compounds, effectively stopping the cycle and decreasing the patient's discomfort and pain.

Digestive enzymes: If a pet is having trouble digesting her food, she won't reap the maximum benefit of her diet or its supplements. Holistic veterinarians often suggest adding digestive enzymes to a pet's food. Older pets, in particular, sometimes lose some of their ability to digest their food and absorb necessary nutrients. Since many arthritic pets are geriatric, digestive enzymes can play a major role in the success of a holistic treatment plan for arthritis.

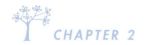 D- L-phenylalanine: D- L-phenylalanine is an amino acid, which is a building block of protein. Normally, the body makes endorphins, or morphinelike substances, and immediately starts tearing them down. D- L-phenylalanine blocks this breakdown process, so it indirectly helps relieve pain by prolonging the effect of the body's own painkillers. D- L-phenylalanine also helps improve muscle strength.

Omega-3 fatty acids: Along with omega-6 fatty acids, omega-3 fatty acids are considered to be the essential fatty acids of the body. Researchers believe that the ratio of omega-3 to omega-6 is what decreases inflammation. One way holistic veterinarians attempt to get the ratio right is through supplementation.

THERAPY #6
MASSAGE THERAPY

Massage therapists perform skilled massage on animals to provide comfort; increase circulation, flexibility, and motility; decrease muscle spasms; and allow muscles and tissues to heal more efficiently—all of which are crucial to the arthritic patient. Additionally, many holistic practitioners believe massage therapy can go beyond musculoskeletal benefits, and studies indicate that massage can reduce acute and chronic pain, improve muscle tone, reduce posttraumatic headache, reduce swelling, and decrease blood pressure and heart rate.

Though massage sounds harmless, therapists warn that massage can release toxins and lactic acid from the muscles. If the buildup in the muscles is severe, the sudden release could be detrimental to the animal's kidneys and liver. A complete blood workup is recommended before a massage to avoid potential complications—especially in geriatric patients. In addition, massage given to animals often must be gentler than given to people.

THERAPY #7
FLOWER ESSENCES

Flower essences are made from extractions of fresh flowers collected in pristine habitats. These essences are potentized medicines, which are remedies that have been diluted and shaken many times (sometimes hundreds of times) to produce substances that are more powerful than if they had been just diluted without shaking. They were developed in the early 1900s by British physician Dr. Edward Bach. Bach's theory was that the disease process begins within an animal as a mental/emotional defect and surfaces with disease symptoms. The flower essences were developed to treat the patient's mental and emotional state. They come in liquid form and can be added to a pet's water (in a bowl) or given orally (directly to a pet). The exact mechanics of how the essences actually alter or improve a patient's mental/emotional state is not known, and there are no scientific studies documenting the effectiveness of flower remedies. Most evidence has come from case studies. The clinical results of flower-essence use have been positive enough that many holistic veterinarians recommend this approach to their clients.

Today there are many manufacturers of flower essences (some with more quality control than others). For a pet suffering from arthritis, one flower-essence combination that is commonly recommended is Rescue Remedy. This combination of cherry plum, clematis, impatiens, rockrose, and star-of-Bethlehem flower essences is frequently used to comfort, calm, and reassure distressed animals.

What You Can Do at Home

In addition to receiving regular holistic care
from an experienced veterinarian, you can
comfort your arthritic pet at home by providing
holistic care. Obviously, the treatments that
require training such as acupuncture, homeopathy, chiropractic, and herbal medicine should
not be attempted by you, a lay person, but
there are many things you can do to boost
the health of your pet, as well as decrease
his pain significantly.

Caring for your arthritic pet involves
paying attention to the animal's comfort.
For example, one of the first things you

should do for your pet is make sure he has a comfortable bed. There are orthopedic beds with special pads that distribute your pet's weight better than a regular pet bed. With a heavy pet, such as a giant dog, this weight distribution can be particularly critical; but an arthritic cat benefits from proper bedding just as much as a heavier animal. If you make your pet's bed yourself, make sure the padding isn't too deep because that would make it difficult for an arthritic animal to rise.

Also, take a good look at your home and yard and re-evaluate it for a pet who has trouble moving. Can your pet comfortably reach his food? You might consider elevating food and water bowls. Where do you keep your pet's bed? Is it on the ground floor, or does your pet have to jump up or climb stairs to reach a favorite sleeping spot? With an arthritic cat, be sure to consider the litter box. How well can your cat climb in and out? You may want to consider providing your cat with a flatter pan-style box. Another problem can be slick floors. Your pet may need better traction in his living areas.

Remember to pay attention to your pet's mental/ emotional condition, as well. Many diseases are thought to worsen if the patient is suffering from stress. A change in routine is enough to stress your pet or make him increasingly despondent. Many holistic practitioners believe that a pet's immune system is heightened if the animal is happy. So try to avoid situations that stress your pet.

Keep a careful eye on your pet and report any significant changes in your pet's health to your veterinarian immediately. Also, don't assume that because your pet shows signs of arthritic pain that he has arthritis. Early intervention is key to the success of treating arthritic patients. Unless your veterinarian makes the diagnosis of arthritis, it may not be arthritis. There are many curable diseases that cause arthritis-like symptoms. Make sure you confirm your suspicions and seek professional treatment.

DIET

Without the proper nutritional building blocks, a healthy pet cannot maintain healthy bones, ligaments, cartilage, tendons, muscles, and joint fluids. His immune system is also weakened. Now, consider the fact that your pet is not 100 percent healthy (because he has arthritis) and has nutritional needs in addition to what is normally required. Without an appropriately enhanced diet, your pet's ability to fight the progression of arthritis will be greatly decreased.

Elderly patients may have an increased need for certain nutrients, along with a decrease in the ability to absorb them. So to give your pet a fighting edge, it is critical that

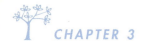

he eat properly. One of the first treatments a holistic veterinarian may suggest is a change in your pet's diet.

Home-Prepared Meals

If you have the time, energy, and ability to feed your pet freshly prepared meals that meet your veterinarian's specifications each day, it is the best way to provide your pet with the exact nutrients he needs without introducing any harmful chemicals or synthetic food preservatives. Preparing a meal of meat, raw vegetables, bonemeal, vitamins, digestive enzymes, and dietary supplements every day, however, is not easy. This type of food preparation demands planning, commitment, and patience in order to create a meal that is beneficial to your pet. If you have a busy schedule, preparing home meals for your pet may not be a viable option.

For those of you who are game to the idea, you will need to work closely with your veterinarian to establish a healthful diet for your arthritic pet. For background information, read *The Holistic Guide for a Healthy Dog* by Wendy Volhard and Kerry Brown, D.V.M., or *It's for the Animals Cookbook* by Helen McKinnon. If you are a cat owner, keep in mind that a cat's protein requirements are quite different from a dog's, so following a recipe for a dog will not suffice for your cat. For example, cats require some animal-origin supplements such as vitamin A and fish oil, not beta-carotene and flax oil as are commonly used in dog meals. Also, realize that the recipes are designed to provide for your pet's needs. Never leave out any ingredients or change their proportions, unless you're absolutely sure it's okay for your pet. If you have questions, always consult with your veterinarian.

If your pet is allergic to some meats—or you want to create a vegetarian meal—proceed with great caution and under the strict supervision of your veterinarian. Cats require higher levels of protein (than dogs do) with a vitamin and amino acid mix found in meats—not plants. Creating the correct mix through a nonmeat diet can be extremely difficult and usually is not recommended (without extensive supplementation with animal-origin foods). Dogs are carnivorous mammals (who happen to include some plant material in their diet) and in a natural environment would eat a meat-based diet along with herbs such as dandelion, Saint-John's-wort, and others. Everything about a cat's and a dog's metabolism is structured around eating meat. If your pet is allergic to one type of meat, you may want to try different kinds before feeding him a strictly nonmeat diet.

While on the subject of allergies, some practitioners believe that allergens can antagonize arthritis. If your pet has a sensitivity to a known allergen, avoid it in the pet's diet. Though not necessarily allergens, food from plants in

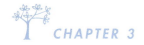

the nightshade family, such as potatoes and tomatoes, can make arthritis worse.

If you choose to purchase your pet's foods, avoid products containing ethoxyquin preservatives, as well as BHA, BHT, nitrates, and nitrites. Feeding foods with these chemicals over a long period may be harmful. Keep in mind that if you feed foods without these preservatives, the food will have a much shorter shelf life. Check expiration or recommended purchase dates before purchasing foods. Also, keep store-bought food in a truly airtight container to maintain freshness. Do not feed your pet rancid or rank-smelling foods—throw them out or return them.

MONITORING WEIGHT AND EXERCISE

Pay attention to your pet's weight. The more your pet weighs, the more stress is placed on his joints. More stress equals more pain and more degeneration. This does not mean you should starve, underfeed, or restrict your pet's necessary nutrients in any way, though. To help slow the degeneration process, you should make sure your pet is at his optimal weight: not too fat and not too skinny.

Keeping an arthritic pet at an optimal weight can be a challenge. Because of aching joints, your pet's regular romping may be severely curtailed. Without frequent exercise, your pet may gain weight more easily. Your veterinarian may suggest feeding your pet a low-fat diet to help compensate for this.

Though your pet may not be particularly thrilled with the idea of exercising his arthritic joints, moderate and gentle exercise is of great benefit. Exercise keeps the joints mobile and strengthens the muscles surrounding the joint, which provides stronger support to the affected area.

The key to exercising your pet is in the words *moderate* and *gentle*. Moderate is not taking your dog hunting all day. Gentle is not asking your cat to repeatedly leap or climb to reach a toy. The best form of exercise is swimming. Swimming allows the arthritic joints a full range of motion and builds muscles without putting any weight on the joints. Of course, a daily swim may not be possible for many dog owners (and too stressful for cats and their owners). If you cannot take your pet swimming, then consider low-intensity walks or slow range-of-motion physical therapy. If you have a cat, you may have to be more creative in designing "walks" or exercise for him, but if your cat tends to follow you from room to room or can be enticed with a tidbit, take advantage of these opportunities.

HOT AND COLD TREATMENTS

Heat is effective and comforting treatment for pets who suffer from arthritis for a long period of time. If your pet's

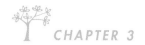

joints are painful and swollen most of the time (not just from flare-ups), heat therapy will allow you to relieve pain, increase blood circulation to the joint and surrounding muscles, and relax muscle spasms. A hot-water bottle wrapped in a towel is good for many large dogs; a lighter, smaller version would be more appropriate for a small dog or a cat.

If your pet is a new sufferer of arthritis (within a year) and has acute swelling in a joint, he may benefit from the application of an occasional cold pack to the affected joint. Be careful with applying a cold pack since a little bit of cold goes a long way. In fact, five minutes of application should be plenty. Anything beyond five minutes might produce negative effects by decreasing the blood circulation to the joint and even perhaps damaging tissues. A good method for making sure you don't accidentally overdo your cold application is to use a sealed freezer bag of frozen corn or peas. The little vegetables are easier to apply than a brick of ice, they are lightweight, and they thaw before they create any problems for your pet. (If you are making home-prepared meals for your pet, you might chop up vegetables that are to be included in your pet's daily meals and freeze them in bags for this purpose.)

If your pet protests either the hot or cold treatments, don't force the issue.

MASSAGE

Taking pets to professional massage therapists is the optimal option, but even if pets are getting regular massages, therapists often ask owners to perform simple massages at home on a daily basis between office visits. Most often, this is a gentle massage given to the pet's neck, shoulders, and lower back. If you're interested in getting the technique right, ask your massage therapist or veterinarian to show you how he or she wants you to work on your pet.

TTouch

Though TTouch is not a true form of massage, this gentle modality invented by Linda Tellington-Jones has been found to relax muscle spasms and the pets themselves. For more information on how to perform this therapy, owners can ask a veterinarian who is skilled in TTouch to give them some pointers. Owners can also read Tellington-Jones's book *The Tellington TTouch: A Revolutionary Natural Method to Train and Care for Your Favorite Animal.*

ACUPRESSURE

Acupressure is a close cousin to acupuncture. The difference is that acupressure doesn't use needles. Acupressure uses finger pressure on specific areas to unblock meridians of energy, which in turn release endorphins that help

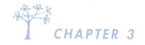

relieve pain and strengthen an animal—both physically and mentally.

Cheryl Schwartz's book *Four Paws, Five Directions* is an excellent resource for learning acupressure, but it would be even better to have hands-on training. Most holistic veterinarians skilled in Asian medicine will be more than happy to show you what acupressure points benefit your pet's condition, as well as teach you how to perform acupressure.

EDUCATE YOURSELF

Empower yourself with knowledge. The more you know, the more you will understand, and the better you will be able to seek out the best possible care for your pet. New studies and theories are constantly emerging from the field of veterinary medicine. If you stay on top of the emerging treatments in both conventional and complementary veterinary medicine, you will be a much more informed consumer and reap the benefits of this. To get started on learning more about arthritis, refer to the selected bibliography for a list of books, magazines, journals, and Web sites.

The future

A variety of holistic options is available to help ease a pet's pain as well as slow or perhaps even stop the degenerative process of arthritis. Currently, however, there is no cure for arthritis. As both conventional and holistic practitioners continue to research effective treatments, hopefully we'll continue to progress toward a cure. The conventional scientific community is increasingly considering holistic theories and treatments. An indication of this is a statement issued by the Arthritis Foundation about its plans to place more emphasis in future research on the "improved understanding and manipulation of the immune system" and the use of "naturally occurring substances in the body to intervene and modify the immune response in people with inflammatory forms of arthritis." Also, an increasing number of veterinarians are graduating from acupuncture school. Previously, graduates numbered thirty or so every other year; today there are ninety graduates each year in the U.S., plus ninety graduates every other year in Canada and in Europe. Some veterinary schools are also offering acupuncture courses as part of their elective curriculum.

The use of Ayurvedic herbs, an Eastern Indian practice, is gaining popularity in the U.S., along with the modality's philosophy that there are three body types and that each type requires a unique and different diet to flourish and be healthy.

As holistic therapies become more accepted in the U.S., pet owners may also see a movement toward "whole pet centers" in which multiple holistic therapies are offered under one roof. For example, there is a center in Los Angeles that offers veterinary chiropractic, massage therapy, swimming pools, treadmills, and other services. Centers such as this may become more common in large cities, and holistic practitioners may become more plentiful in even more remote and isolated areas.

RESOURCES FOR
FINDING A HOLISTIC VET

For referrals to holistic veterinarians in your area, or if you would like to receive more information, please consult the following associations:

Academy of Veterinary Homeopathy
751 N.E. 168th Street
c/o Larry Bernstein, V.M.D
North Miami Beach, FL 33162-2427
(305) 652-5372; fax: (305)-653-7244
 e-mail: avh@naturalholistic.com or academy@docb.com

American Holistic Veterinary Medical Association
2214 Old Emmorton Road
Bel Air, MD 21015
(410) 569-0795

American Veterinary Chiropractic Association
623 Main Street
Hillsdale, IL 61257
(309) 658-2920; fax: (309) 658-2622

International Association for Veterinary Homeopathy
Susan G. Wynn, D.V.M.
334 Knollwood Lane

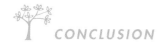

CONCLUSION

Woodstock, GA 30188
(770) 516-5954
 e-mail: swynn@emory.edu

International Veterinary Acupuncture Society
P.O. Box 1478
Longmont, CO 80502
(303) 682-1167; fax: (303) 682-1168
e-mail: IVASOffice@aol.com

Much of the research and information on natural medicine comes from a variety of sources that can be difficult to find. While the amount of written research is growing, a lot of the information still can be found only in unpublished sources. In addition to using the conventional sources such as books, magazines, and veterinary journals, the author interviewed holistic and conventional veterinarians and researched several unpublished sources, including news releases and articles from the Internet. Following are sources in which you can find more information on arthritis.

Books and Magazines

Allport, Richard. *Heal Your Dog the Natural Way*. New York: Howell Book House, 1997.

Altman, R.D., D.D. Dean, O.E. Muiz, and D.S. Howell. "Therapeutic Treatment of Canine Osteoarthritis with Glucosaminoglycan Polysulfuric Acid Ester." *Arthritis and Rheum* 32, no. 10 (Oct. 1989).

American Veterinary Medical Association. "Pet Owners Tune to Alternative Therapies." *Dog World,* 83, no. 11: 52–53.

Basko, I.J. "To Shark or Not to Shark? That is the Question?" *Journal of the American Holistic Veterinary Medical Association* 14, no. 2: 27.

Cargill, John C. and Susan Thorpe-Vargas. "Stirring the Food Pot with Supplements." *Dog World,* 83, no. 11: 20–25.

Dustman, Karen Dale. "Relieving Arthritis Naturally." *Natural Pet,* August 1996, 26–30, 32, 71.

Frazier, Anitra. *The New Natural Cat.* New York: E.P. Dutton, 1990.

Gottlieb, Bill. *New Choices in Natural Healing.* Emmaus, PA: Rodale Press, Inc., 1995.

"Herbal Industry Takes to the Lab to Standardize Supplements." *The Virginian-Pilot,* October 13, 1998, A-5.

Jacobs, Jennifer, consulting editor. *The Encyclopedia of Alternative Medicine.* Boston: Journey Editions, 1996.

Kastner, Mark and Hugh Burroughs. *Alternative Healing: The Complete A–Z Guide to Over 160 Alternative Therapies.* Aukland, New Zealand: Halcyon Publishing, 1993.

Lauerman, J. "Inflammation Easers." *New Age Journal,* January/February 1996, 108, 110.

Lewis, L.D. "Nutrition for Recovery." *Veterinary Forum,* January 1996, 58–59.

Manning, A. "Can Nutrient Combo Really Work Wonders on Arthritis?" *USA Today,* Health, March 17, 1998.

Manning, A. "Drugs Battle Cause of Arthritis." *USA Today,* Health, March 17, 1998.

McKinnon, Helen. *It's for the Animals Cookbook.* Clinton, NJ: CSA, Inc., 1995.

Morton, Michael and Mary Morton. *Five Steps to Selecting the Best Alternative Care: A Guide to Complementary and Integrative Health Care.* Novato, CA: New World Library, 1997.

Moser, E.A. "Antioxidant Vitamins in Canine Nutrition." *Veterinary Technician,* Nov/Dec 1994, 587–589.

Pisetsky, D.S. and S.F. Trien. *The Duke University Medical Center Book of Arthritis.* Durham: Duke University Press, 1995.

Pitcairn, Richard, D.V.M. and Susan Hubble Pitcairn. *Dr. Pitcairn's Complete Guide to Natural Health for Dogs and Cats,* Emmaus, PA: Rodale Press, Inc., 1995.

Puotinen, CJ. *The Encyclopedia of Natural Pet Care.* New Canaan, CT: Keats Publishing, 1998.

"The Role of Gelatin-Based Dietary Supplements in Maintaining Joint Health" *Medical Sciences Bulletin,* no. 248–249, May/June 1998.

Schoen, Allen M., D.V.M., M.S. and Susan Wynn, eds. *Complementary and Alternative Veterinary Medicine Principles and Practice.* St. Louis: Mosby, 1998.

Schwartz, Cheryl, D.V.M. *Four Paws, Five Directions.* Berkeley, CA: Celestial Arts, 1996.

Sobel, D. and A.C. Klein. *Arthritis: What Works.* New York: St. Martins, 1992.

Stein, P. *Natural Health Care for Your Dog.* Hauppage, NY: Barron's, 1997.

Tellington-Jones, Linda. *The Tellington TTouch: A Revolutionary Natural Method to Train and Care for Your Favorite Animal.* New York: Penguin USA, 1995.

Tengerdy, R. "The Role of Vitamin E in Immune Response and Disease Prevention." *Annals NY Academy of Science* 587 (1990): 24–33.

Volhard, Wendy and Kerry Brown, D.V.M. *The Holistic Guide for a Healthy Dog.* New York: Howell Book House, 1995.

Walker, Joan H. "Chiropractic Pet Care." *Natural Pet,* August 1996, 42–48.

Walker, Joan H. "Energy-based Therapies." *Natural Pet,* April 1997, 70–83.

Watts, D.L. *Trace Elements and Other Essential Nutrients.* Dallas: Watts Publications, 1995.

Werback, Melvyn R. *Botanical Influences on Illness.* Tarzana, CA: Third Line Press, 1994.

Werbach, M.R. *Nutritional Influences on Illness: A Sourcebook of Clinical Research.* New Canaan, CT: Keats Publishing, 1996.

Internet and Other Sources

"Arthritis Fact Sheet." *Arthritis Foundation,* 1998. www.arthritis.org/resource/fs/arthritis.shtml

"Arthritis Foundation's Recommendations for Preventing or Reducing the Effects of Arthritis." *Arthritis Foundation,* September 23, 1998. www.arthritis.org.

"Arthritis in Dogs: Pain Relief Options Expanding," Kansas State University News Services, May 28, 1997.

"Arthritis Research." *Arthritis Foundation.* 1998. www.arthritis.org

Beinfield, H. and E. Korngold. "Chinese Medicine: How It Works." *Health World Online.* 1991. www.healthy.net/library/

DeCava, J., *The Real Truth About Vitamins and Antioxidants: Health Science Series,* no. 5. Brentwood Academic Press, 1996.

Foster, Race, D.V.M. "Arthritis and Pets: What You Can Do," *Doctors Foster and Smith, Inc.* ©1997–98. www.drsfostersmith.com

Fuess, T.A. "Arthritis in Cats and Dogs." University of Illinois, College of Veterinary Medicine, *Pet Column,* February 9, 1998.

Gelber, A.C., "Can Vitamins Slow Arthritis?" John Hopkins News, *InteliHealth,* John Hopkins Medical Institutions, December 12, 1997. www.intelihealth.com

"Glucosamine Sulfate and Chondroitin Sulfate." *Arthritis Foundation, Memo,* February 20, 1997. www.arthritis.org

"Guidelines for Alternative and Complementary Veterinary Medicine." *AVMA Policy Statements and Guidelines,* 1996.

Hobbs, Christopher. "An Outline of the History of Herbalism: An Overview and Literature Resource List." *Health World Online,* 1996. www.healthy.net/library/

Hoffman, David L. "Rheumatoid Arthritis." *Health World Online,* 1998. healthy.net/library/

Hoffman, David L. "Inflammation and Arthritis." *Health World Online,* 1998. healthy.net/library/

Hoffman, David L. "Osteoarthritis." *Health World Online,* 1998. healthy.net/library/

Janson, M. "Arthritis." *Health World Online,* 1996. healthy.net/library/

Kaslof, L.J. "Your Pet's Emotional Health." *Health World Online,* 1996. www.healthy.net/library/

"Medical Benefits of Massage Are Still Unclear." *Pennsylvania State College of Health and Human Development News Service,* September 15, 1998.

"Osteoarthritis Fact Sheet." *Arthritis Foundation,* 1998. www.arthritis.org

"Rheumatoid Arthritis Fact Sheet." *Arthritis Foundation,* 1998. www.arthritis.org

Rivera, Pedro Luis. "Antioxidants: The Missing Link for the Treatment of Degenerative Processes." *Proceedings of the 1996 AHVMA Annual Conference,* 142–147.

Rivera, Pedro Luis "Introduction to Veterinary Chiropractic." *Proceedings of the 1996 AHVMA Annual Conference, 1996:* 140–141.

Rivera, Pedro Luis. "Joint Fluid Supplements and Organ Therapy for Cartilage Problems." *American Holistic Veterinary Medical Association (AHVMA) Proceedings, 1995:* 105–108.

Rivera, Pedro Luis, presenter, "Bach Flower Remedies." *Proceedings of the Midwest Holistic Veterinary Conference, 1996:* 68–75.

Tellington-Jones, Linda. *Tellington Touch for Happier Cats.* 60 min. Silma Delta Research, 1998. Videocassette.

Tellington-Jones, Linda. *Tellington Touch for Happier Dogs.* 60 min. Silma Delta Research, 1997. Videocassette.

Theodosakis, Jason, M.D. "Dr. Theo's Q&A About Arthritis." and "Dr. Theo's Q&A About the Treatment Program." *Dr. Theo Online,* 1998. www.drtheo.com

Theodasakis, Jason, M.D. "The Medical Evidence." *Dr. Theo Online,* 1998. www.drtheo.com

Ullman, Dana. "A Condensed History of Homeopathy." *Health World Online,* 1995. www.healthy.net/library/

Ullman, Dana. "Arthritis." excerpted from "The One Minute (or so) Healer." *Health World Online,* 1995. www.healthy.net/library/

Ullman, Dana. "Homeopathic Medicines for Arthritis." *Health World Online,* 1995. www.healthy.net/library/

"Unproven Remedies Fact Sheet." *Arthritis Foundation,* 1998. www.arthritis.org

"What are Flower Remedies?" *Health World Online,* 1998. www.healthy.net/library/

"What is Holistic Veterinary Medicine?" *American Holistic Veterinary Medical Association Web-site,* 1998. www.altvetmed.com

Wynn, Susan G., D.V.M. "Arthritis." *American Holistic Veterinary Medical Association Web-site,* 1996. www.altvetmed.com

ABOUT THE AUTHOR

Joan Hustace Walker has been writing professionally since 1984. She is a member of the Authors Guild, the American Society of Journalists and Authors, the Dog Writers Association of America, the Cat Writers Association, and the Society of Environmental Journalists. She formerly served as a contributing editor for *Natural Pet* magazine. An award-winning writer specializing in animals, health, and environmental issues, Walker writes for both general and technical audiences. She has had more than 150 articles published by a variety of magazines and has written several books. She lives in Virginia.

ABOUT THE VETERINARIAN

Dr. Nancy Scanlan graduated from University of California, Davis, in 1970. She has used nutritional therapy since her senior year there. She has been certified in veterinary acupuncture since 1988 and has taught animal health and animal science for ten years. Dr. Scanlan regularly writes articles for various pet-related magazines. She currently practices holistic-only medicine in California, using acupuncture, nutritional therapy, Chinese and Western herbs, trigger point therapy, and chiropractic. If you are interested in getting in touch with Dr. Scanlan, contact the American Holistic Veterinary Medical Association.

For more about natural pet care, look for *Natural Dog* and *Natural Cat* magazines at pet stores and selected newsstands.

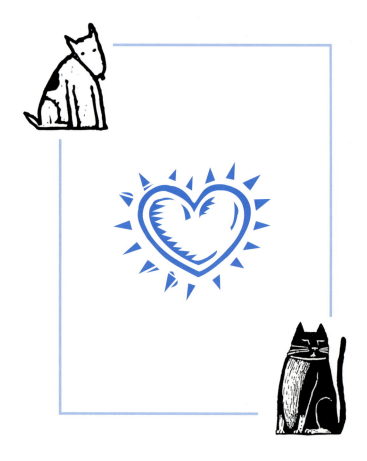